Every Page

The Day One Guide to Your Period

EveryPage

The Day One Guide to Your Period

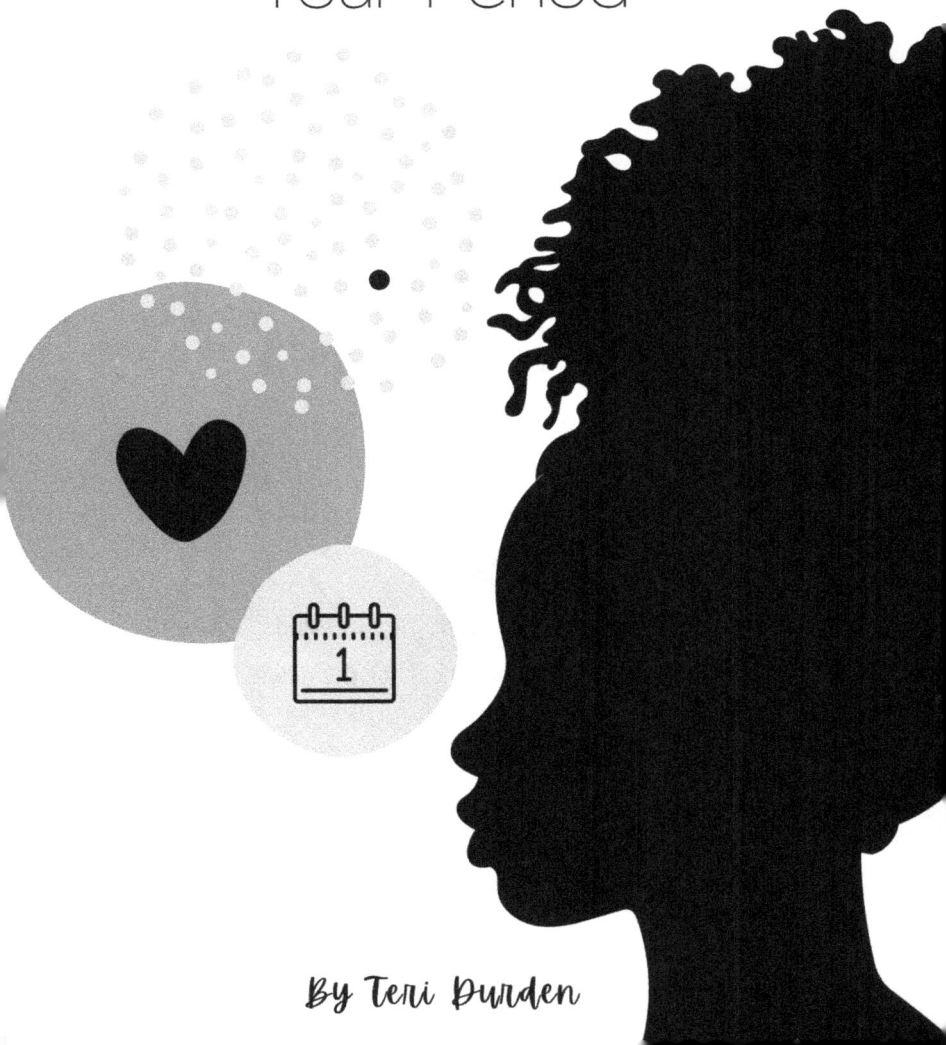

By Teri Durden

Written by Teri Durden

Copyright © 2022 by Teri Durden

Cover Design & Illustrations by Teri Durden

ISBN 979-8-218-43058-0

For the girl in need of a hand to hold as she grows into
the fearfully and wonderfully made
woman God created her to be.
You got this.

TABLE OF
CONTENTS

This book is meant to be fun, educational, and informative.

It is not medical advice.

Menstruating girls and women can use this book to look for clues to manage their menstrual symptoms; however, it is not meant to help diagnose or treat menstrual disorders.

For testing, a diagnosis, or treatment, please seek out a medical professional.

Teri Durden is certified by the Institute for Menstrual Health.

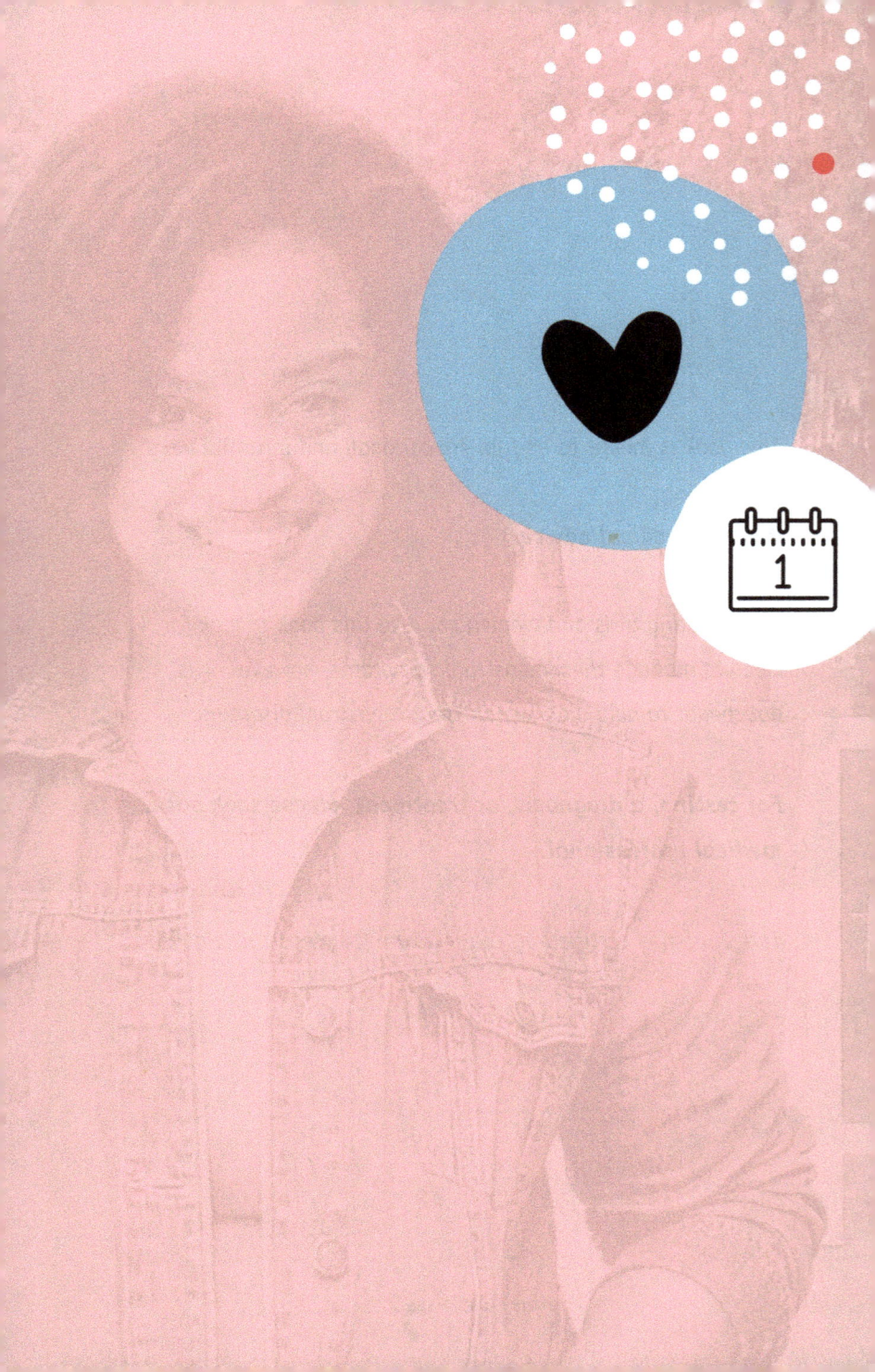

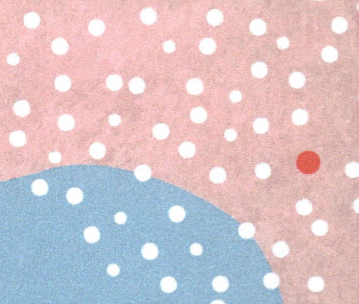

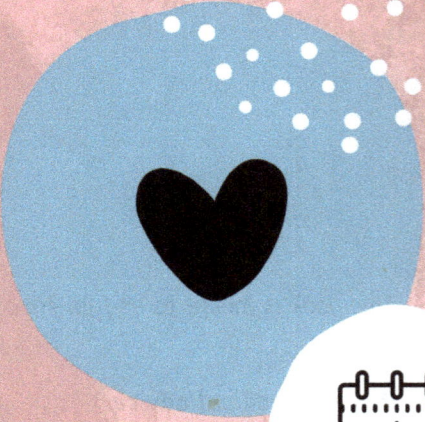

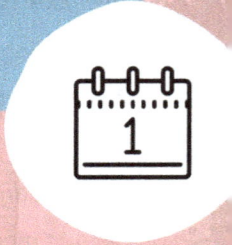

Don't Skip This Section

My name is Teri.

I was nine years old when I got my first period, but I didn't tell anyone until Day 2.

Why? Partly because I wanted to be sure, but I also felt shame and embarrassment.

I don't want that to be your story.

I want you to have all the information and support you need to have a healthy view of your period and everything that comes with it, even if Day 1 hasn't arrived just yet.

If you're a pre-teen or a teenage girl, every page of this book was written with you in mind, so dive right in.

Read through this book once, then again and again. Refer back to it often – not only for yourself, but for your fellow sisters and friends.

Your period is a monthly reminder that your body is sacred and every detail of you matters. Through this book, I hope to shed light on that truth.

Understanding your period in full will open your eyes to new ways to love and respect your body like nothing and no one else.

That love and respect will reflect in your choices.

To the adult women reading this book, please take this message to heart. Celebrate Day 1 with your daughters and granddaughters, nieces and cousins.

Gift them a period kit, throw them a period party, or simply make yourself available to answer their questions!

If you are like me and you walked through Day 1 alone, or if your period came with any physical or emotional pain that followed you through adulthood, please know that I wrote this book for you as well.

Close your eyes, bring that young girl to mind, and tell her she's okay. No matter what's troubling her, she is seen, known, and deeply loved by her Creator; and pain is not her portion.

Accept this book as an invitation to pause, to embrace rest, and to begin healing. Beauty will come from it.

All my best,
Teri

Jesus turned, and seeing her he said, "Take heart, daughter; your faith has made you well."
Matthew 9:22

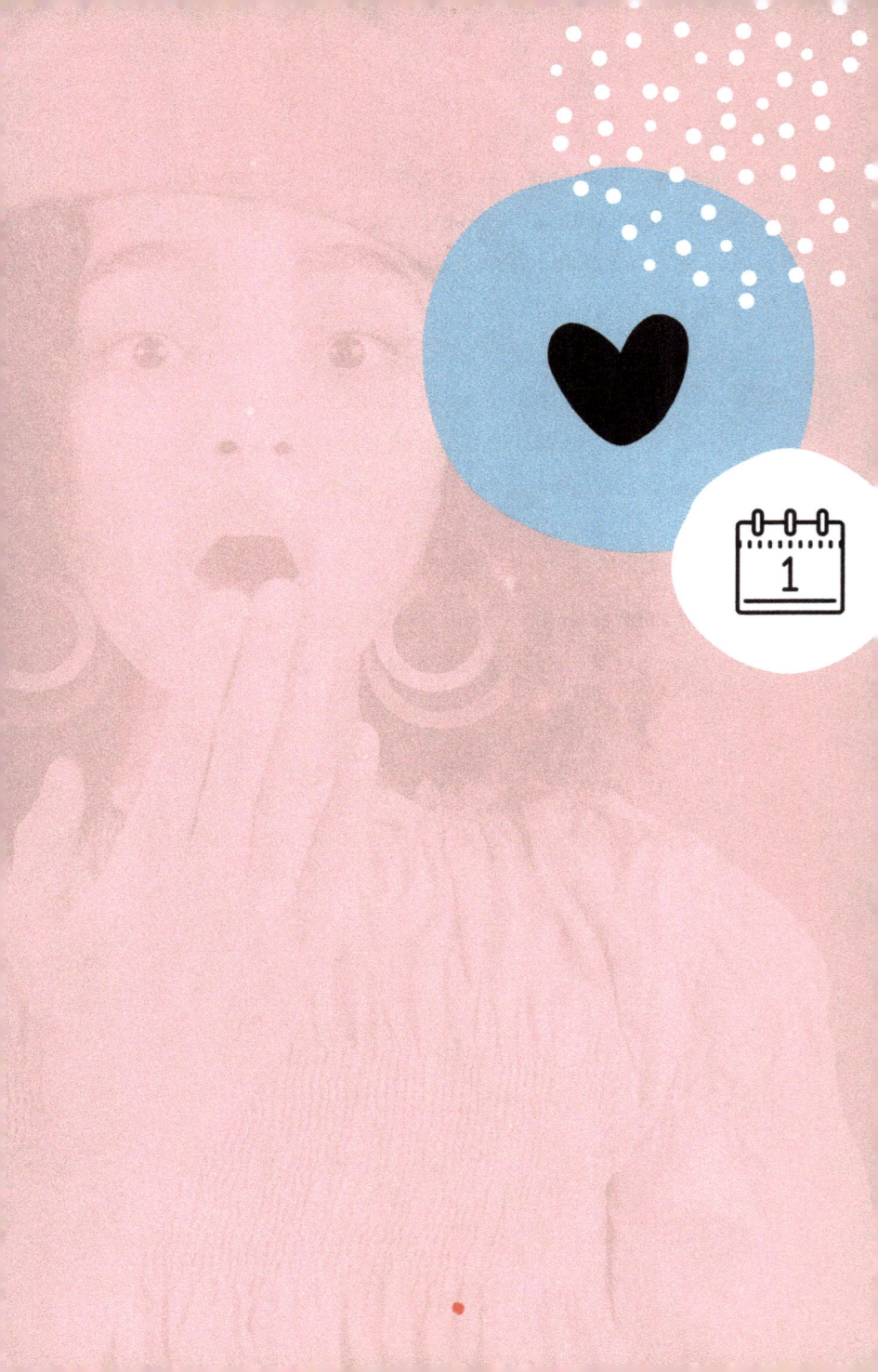

CHAPTER 1

You Got This

Did your period arrive today?

Don't panic. I'm here to help!

First things first, take a deep breath and contact someone you trust. Let them know that you started your period and you need a pad.

If that person is an adult – like a parent, teacher, or school nurse – then chances are, they won't need an explanation and can provide assistance.

If it's a close friend, that's okay, too!

Not at home or at school? No access to a pad? Not a problem.

Find the nearest restroom, then grab some toilet paper and gently wrap a small wad around your hand. It should be thick enough to be absorbent, but small enough to fit comfortably in your underwear.

Before you pull up your undies, use another piece of toilet paper to dry up any period blood stains. If they're already dry – perfect!

Your handmade pad should hold you over until you find a real one.

Is there a visible spot on the back of your clothes? Don't worry. That will come out with soap and cold water, or a little stain remover.

If you don't have a change of clothes, find a pullover, a jacket, or a long-sleeve shirt and wrap it around your waist. If you don't have any of those things nearby, then don't sweat it.

Keep your cool and focus on finding help. No one is looking as closely as you might think.

Own those spots and keep it moving.

You got this.

Once you are at home, and hopefully in possession of a few pads, wash up and put on a fresh one.

Now get cozy because we have so much to talk about!

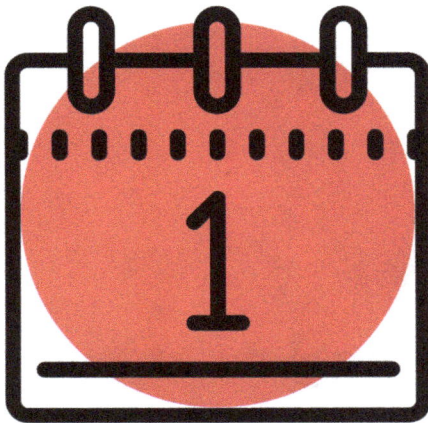

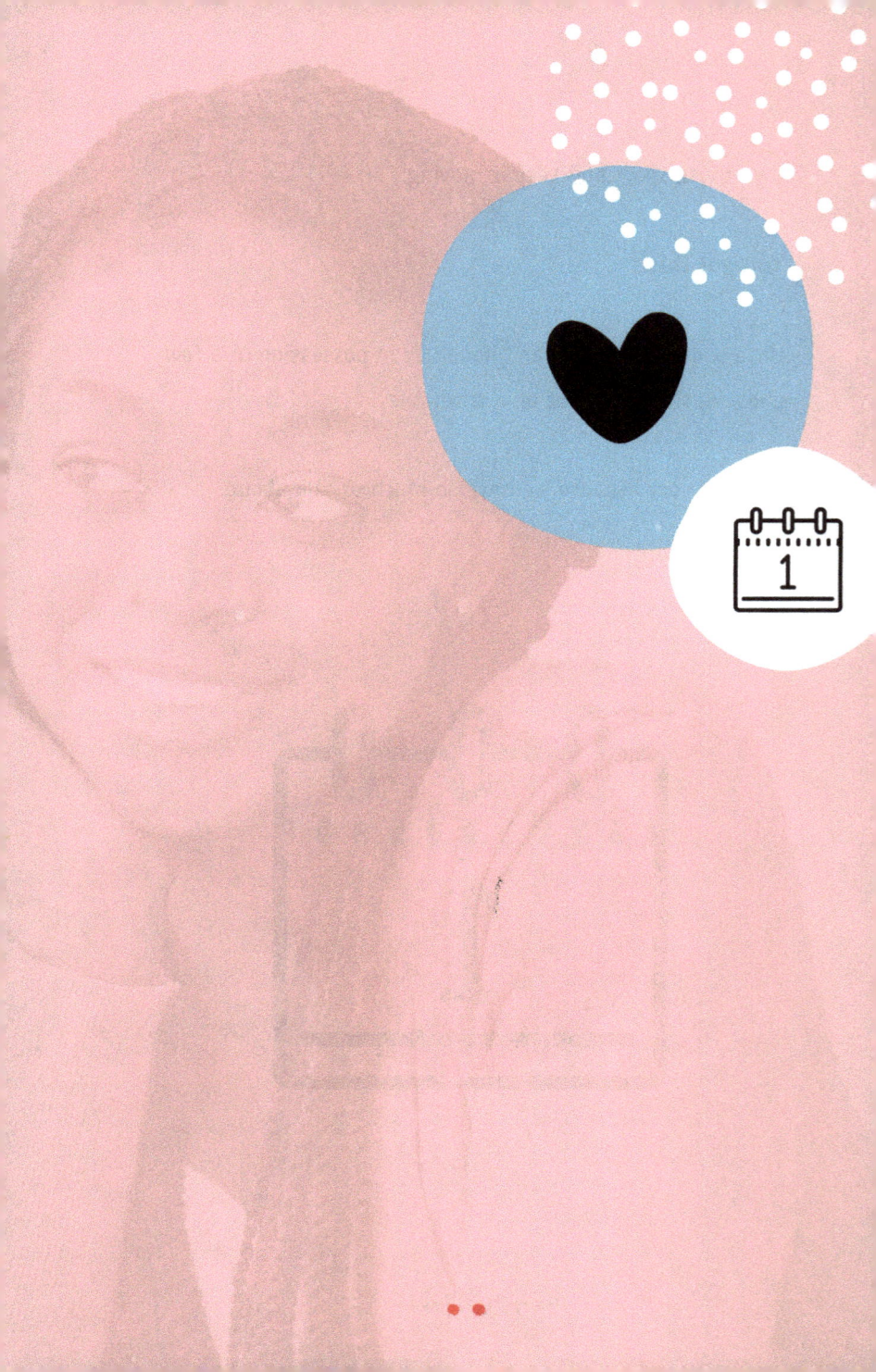

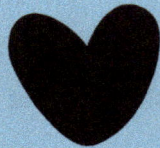

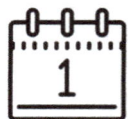

CHAPTER 2

Tune Into Your Body

How are you feeling?

Grab a journal or a sheet of paper and write it down.

Notice how you feel physically and emotionally. If any questions or concerns come to mind, write those down, too.

Make these daily check-ins a habit - even between periods.

Call it your period journal or your menstrual diary.

For the next 3 to 7 days, pay attention to your needs. Notice how your period blood flow changes and how frequently you need to change your pad.

You may find yourself wanting to sleep a little longer, shower more often, or be alone. This is totally normal. You may not notice anything but the pad. That's normal, too!

No matter what feelings arise, know that you are not alone and that I'm cheering you on.

That's right. The start of your period should be celebrated! It marks the beginning of a new chapter in your life where your body is changing in a beautiful way.

Even if you can't see it or feel it, from the inside out, you are blossoming and becoming all you were created to be.

Your body is producing the hormones you need to grow into a strong, healthy, and fearfully created woman (but not overnight!). Everything from your hair and your skin to your heart and your bones is evolving.

Pat yourself on the back and rest well. Days like these are meant to be slower than others.

Keep your period journal close, and don't be afraid to ask questions. The sooner you get answers to those questions, the more confident you will feel as you navigate this new chapter.

Lucky for you, this book is full of answers, so keep reading!

While you're at it, drink plenty of water and eat nourishing foods. As you feel yourself winding down, prepare for a good night's sleep. This will help you reset for Day 2.

In no time, you will start to feel like yourself again. If not, don't worry too much. We will tackle those blues together.

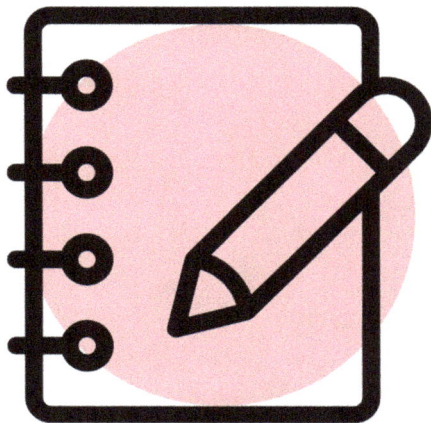

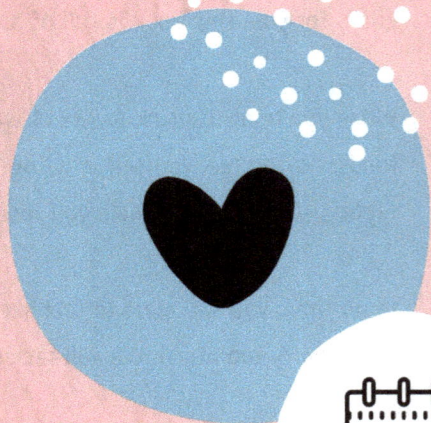

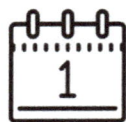

CHAPTER 3

Let's Talk About Hygiene

How do you feel about the pads? Are they absorbent enough? Is the size okay?

Pads are one of many forms of period protection, and it's important to choose the one that's right for you.

Your period protection should not only help minimize leaks, but it should also be comfortable.

This is an important part of your period hygiene!

For starters, you are more than likely using disposable pads that stick to your underwear. These come in a variety of sizes, shapes, and absorbances; and for your convenience, they are available at most drugstores and grocery stores. You can try different brands, but most get the job done.

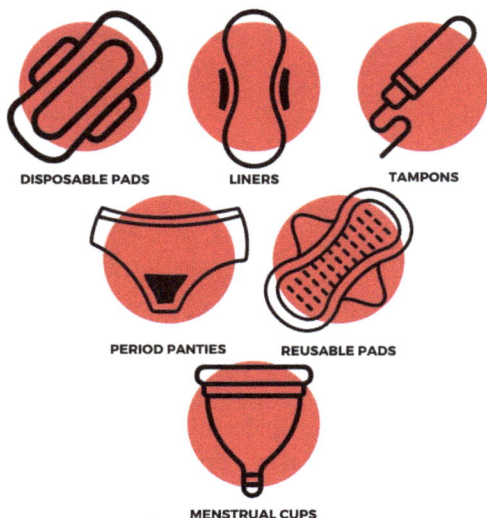

DISPOSABLE PADS　　**LINERS**　　**TAMPONS**

PERIOD PANTIES　　**REUSABLE PADS**

MENSTRUAL CUPS

Many girls start out using disposable pads, and with time, they might incorporate tampons. Like pads, tampons come in different sizes, but they are worn in the opening of the vagina. For extra protection, some girls pair them with a panty liner, which is much smaller than a pad.

As you are figuring out your flow, I recommend using disposable pads. If you play sports, then you may want to give tampons a try, but only when you feel comfortable.

The diagram above shows more examples of period protection to potentially explore at a later time.

Whichever period protection you choose, follow the instructions on the packaging carefully, and be sure to change regularly (every 3 to 4 hours).

Never let a pad or liner fill up with a day's worth of blood, and never leave a tampon in for more than a few hours. This will help minimize potential leaks, odors, and toxicity.

Dispose of your pads by folding them up and wrapping them in toilet paper, then throw them in the trash. Used tampons can be flushed down the toilet, but the tampon applicator (the plastic or cardboard part!) should be thrown in the trash.

Always use clean hands while handling your period protection. Your vaginal area is highly sensitive, so eliminate the possibility of transferring germs or irritants by washing your hands with soap and water.

Before you leave the restroom, look behind you. Is the toilet seat free of red drops or smears? Does the view from the back of your clothes look normal? No bulging pad, no spots, no skirt tucked into your undies by mistake? Are all of your used pads or tampons properly disposed of?

Are your hands and nails clean? If everything looks good, then you're free to go about your day.

If you have a leak, hand wash your underwear with soap and cold water, then hang to dry before throwing them in the laundry.

In case of future accidents, carry an extra pair of undies in your bag, keep plenty of period protection on hand, and make a mental note of where restrooms are wherever you go. It is also acceptable to pack extra clothing.

Shower as normal or as often as you need to; and use a gentle, fragrance-free soap and warm water for cleansing.

When you step out of the shower, you may experience a leak from time to time. Dry off with a dark colored towel. If you don't have one, use what you have to dry your body, then grab some toilet paper or a paper towel to dry between your legs and around your vaginal area.

From there, put on your period protection.

With time, these hygiene habits will come together for you naturally.

There's nothing to be ashamed of when it comes to your period and your period hygiene. This is a learning process, so be kind to yourself and ask for help if needed.

You can resume your normal activities, but keep your period supplies handy and make hygiene a priority. See what to add to your period kit on pages 55–56!

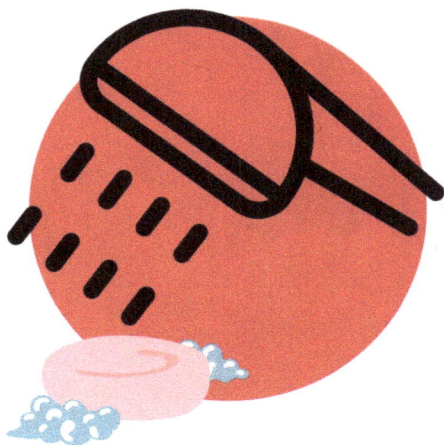

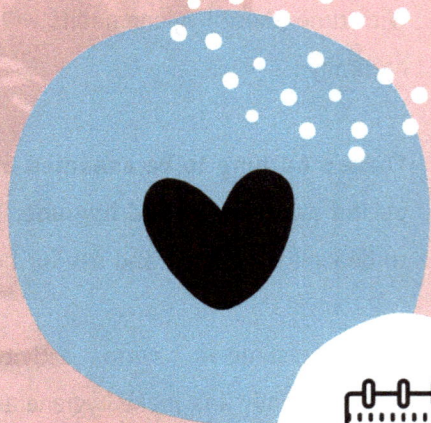

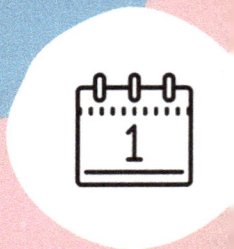

CHAPTER 4

Mark Your Calendar

Let's switch things up and do another activity. Grab a calendar (or flip to page 66!) and place a big dot on the day you first started your period. From there, mark every day that you have your period (or bleed), from start to finish.

A quick warning: don't get duped by a sudden pause in your period! Wear your period protection over the next 3 to 7 days as your body continues to adjust to the change.

Track the start of your period every month - to plan ahead and to get a clear picture of the number of days in your period and your menstrual cycle. That way, you can begin to predict the start of your next period.

For the first 3 to 4 years, period tracking may be challenging as the number of days in your period and your menstrual cycle can change from month to month. This is a sign that your body is still adjusting, so give it time.

A healthy menstrual cycle can be anywhere from 21 to 35 days long, and your period can last anywhere from 3 to 7 days of that cycle. For young girls, however, your menstrual cycle can be up to 45 days long with a period from 2 to 7 days long.

A new cycle begins the first day of your next period.

The diagram below illustrates bleeding days in comparison to non-bleeding days during a menstrual cycle.

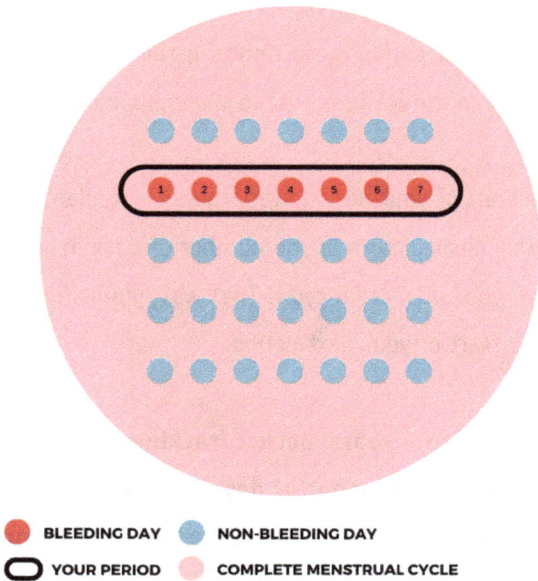

BLEEDING DAY   NON-BLEEDING DAY
YOUR PERIOD   COMPLETE MENSTRUAL CYCLE

On average, my menstrual cycle is 27 to 28 days long. Knowing this helps me to predict when my next period will start. Usually, it lasts for 5 days, so I wear period protection and take notes on how I'm feeling for each of those days.

During this time, I keep my social calendar light and focus on rest and recovery. I also reflect on all the things I want to accomplish after my period.

With time, you will learn to protect this time on your calendar, too.

It's okay to decline invitations, reschedule hangouts with friends, or modify your daily routine to suit the bleeding phase of your cycle. It's only for a short time each month.

A new cycle begins the first day of your next period.

Whether you're using a physical or digital calendar, or even a calendar you created yourself, it's important to not only be aware of when you start your period and how long it lasts, but also if you skip one. If you do happen to skip one, don't worry too much. Keep track of it. Your body is still adjusting.

These monthly rhythms will be a part of your life for the next few decades, so keep a calendar handy. View my sample calendar below, then jump to page 65 for a link to my printable one-year calendar template!

MONTHLY PERIOD CALENDAR (EXAMPLE)

October

S	M	T	W	T	F	S
☹	☹	①	②	③	④	⑤
☺	☺	☺				

Oct 8: I felt a bit sad
Oct 9: I didn't get enough sleep
Oct 11-12: My period flow was heavy

☺ GOOD DAY ☹ NOT-SO-GOOD DAY ⬤ BLEEDING DAY

NOTES

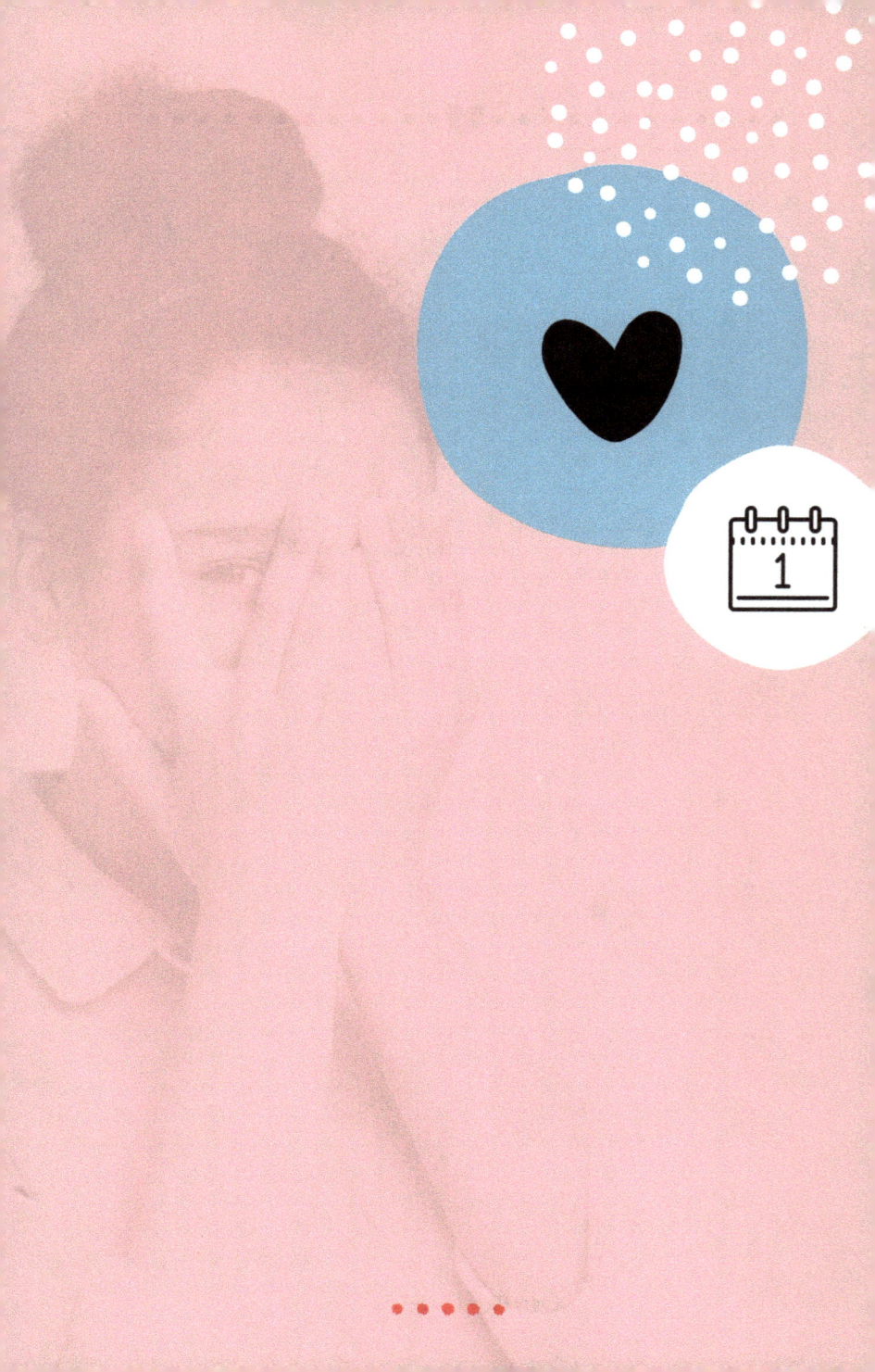

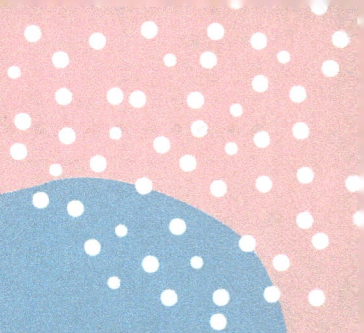

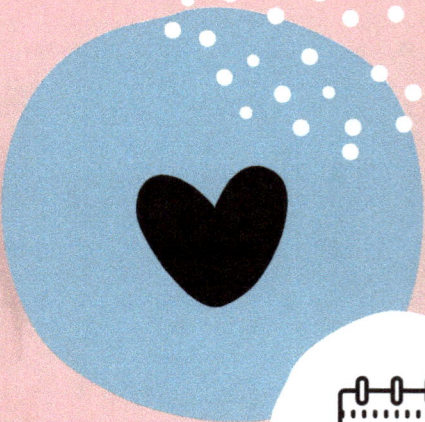

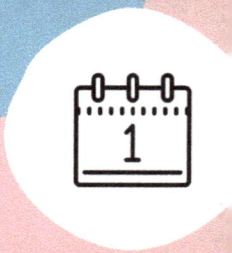

CHAPTER 5

What's This All About?

By now, you are probably wondering what all this bleeding is about. I will try my best to explain in simple terms.

Menstruation

Your first bleed (or menarche) is an important milestone on your journey to womanhood.

To help you on that journey, your body moves through a complete cycle each month to produce the female hormones (estrogen and progesterone) you need to develop into a strong and healthy woman. The 3 to 7 days of that cycle where you bleed is called your period. This is also known as menstruation.

Girls can experience their first bleed anywhere from age 8 to 16, but for many, it comes between ages 12 and 13.

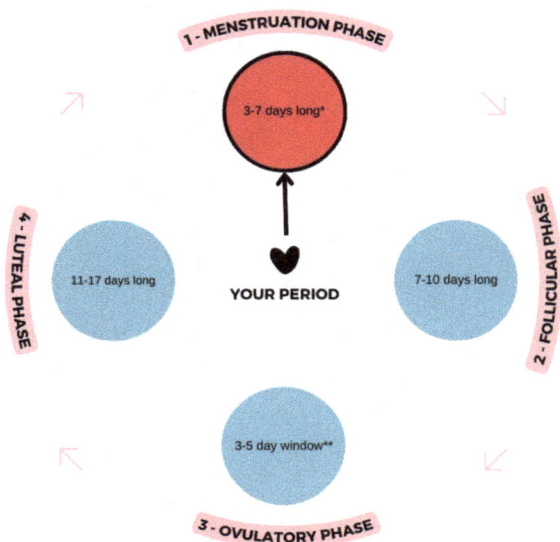

1 - MENSTRUATION PHASE

3-7 days long*

YOUR PERIOD

4 - LUTEAL PHASE

11-17 days long

2 - FOLLICULAR PHASE

7-10 days long

3 - OVULATORY PHASE

3-5 day window**

*This includes Day 1 of your period
**This window includes the days just
before and after ovulation.

The complete cycle, which begins on the first day of your period and ends at the start of your next period, is called your menstrual cycle. For the average woman, it's about 29 days long and includes four phases. (See the diagram above for reference.)

This process not only ensures proper development, but also prepares your body for reproduction. This is how women become pregnant with a baby. At the appropriate time, your parent or guardian can discuss this with you in greater detail. For now, I'll briefly explain the part your body plays in the miracle of life.

Non-Bleeding Follicular, Ovulatory, and Luteal Phases

As a menstruating girl, each month, your body produces a preovulatory follicle that contains one egg. This follicle grows during your follicular phase; then the egg is released from one of your ovaries through a process called ovulation. This is made possible by your hormones. The egg travels down one of your fallopian tubes during your ovulatory phase and implants in your uterus. At that time, the lining of your uterus (or endometrium) becomes thicker. This is a key part of the second half of your cycle!

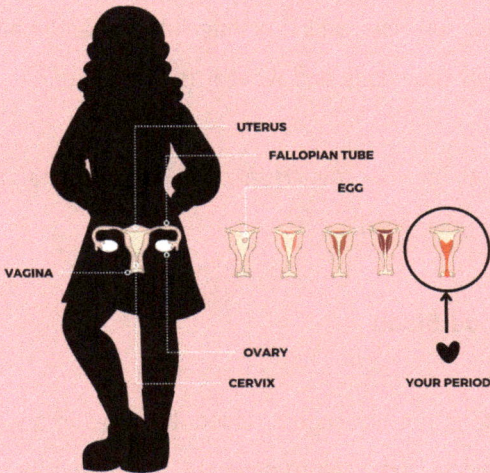

UTERUS
FALLOPIAN TUBE
EGG
VAGINA
OVARY
CERVIX
YOUR PERIOD

The diagram above illustrates how the lining of your uterus thickens to support the egg during your luteal phase.

If the egg is not fertilized, it dissolves; and the lining of your uterus sheds and leaves your body through your vagina. This is why you begin to bleed period blood. You can expect this to happen every month throughout your menstruating years. For most women, those last through their 40s and 50s.

The internal, hormonal changes that happen throughout your menstrual cycle make ovulation (and future pregnancy) possible! **This recurring process is a sign of health in girls and women as it supports our minds and bodies.**

With time, your body (and your mindset) will adjust to these changes; but for now, isn't it wonderful to imagine all that's happening in your body and what it is capable of?

Everything about your menstrual cycle is intentional and working for your good.

About Period Blood

Period blood is not like regular blood. It comes in a wide range of colors, from pink to deep red and brown, but generally, a saturated red color is what you want to see (think rose, ruby, or cherry reds).

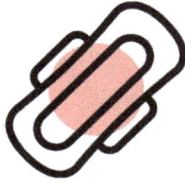

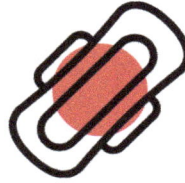

PINK TO BRIGHT REDS

Blood mixed with cervical
fluid that makes it
appear lighter; usually thin
in consistency

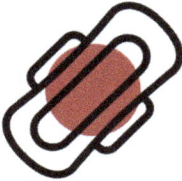

**ROSE, RUBY, AND
CHERRY REDS**

Healthy, saturated
period blood; usually thick
in consistency

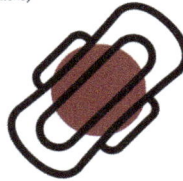

**DEEP PURPLE
TO BROWN**

Slow-moving or old
blood at the beginning or
end of your period

Period blood consists of the uterine lining, red blood cells, and other fluids. For these reasons, healthy period blood has the consistency of maple syrup – not too watery, not too thick, or clumpy.

If you ever notice that your period blood is consistently too light (pink), too thick (think jam), or contains large clumps (the size of a quarter or larger), then talk to your doctor as these can be signs of underlying issues that should be addressed sooner rather than later.

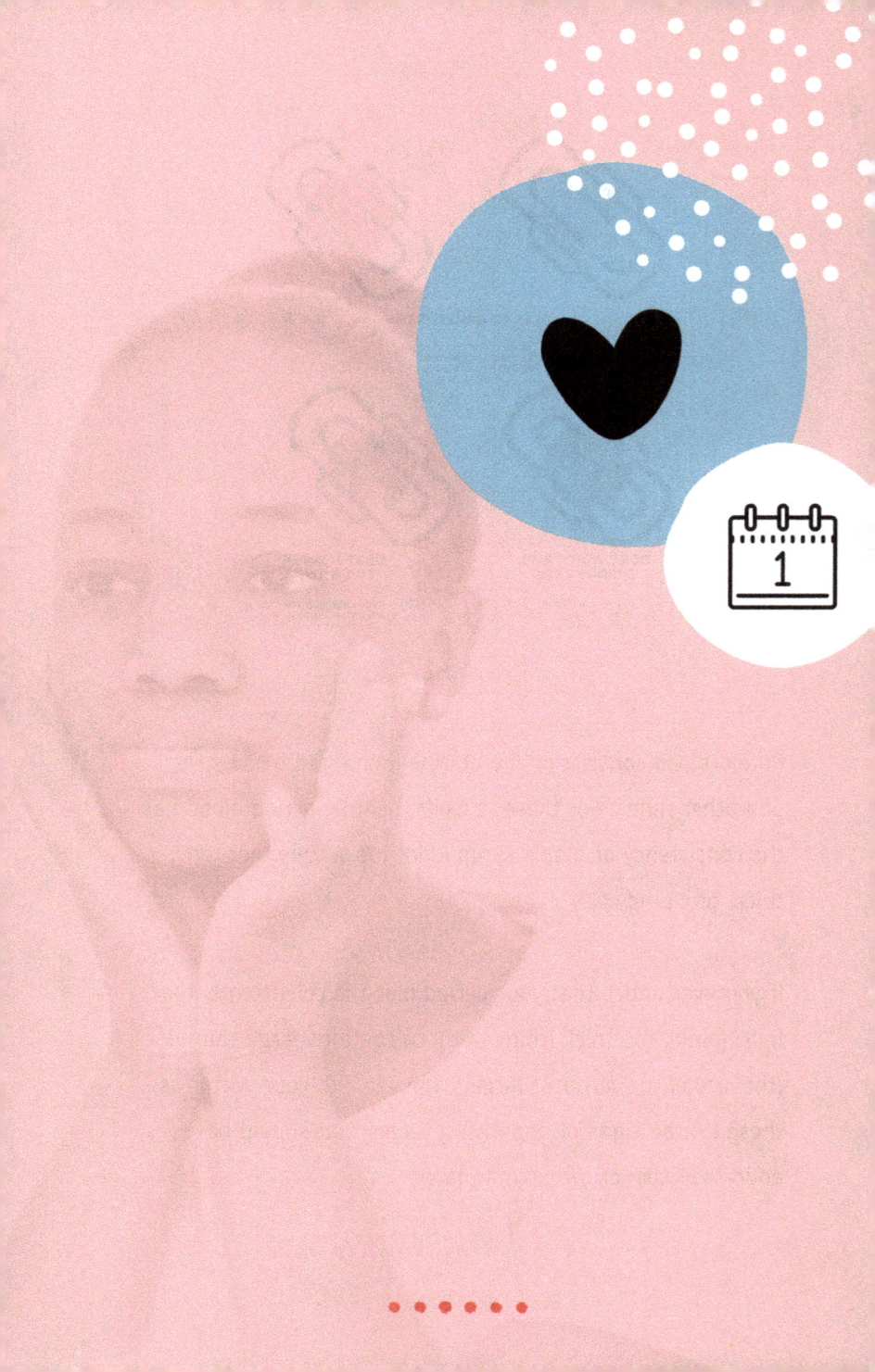

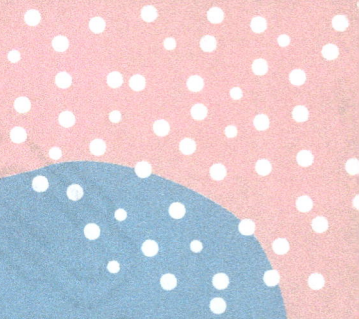

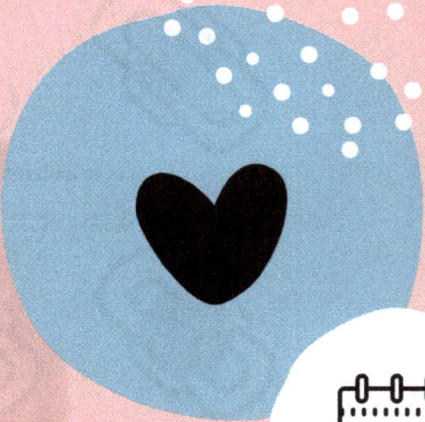

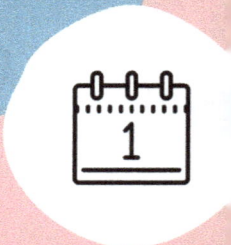

CHAPTER 6

Food & Lifestyle Choices

A big part of your period health is what you eat and drink, and the choices you make daily. That includes when you sleep, how you manage stress, and the types of physical activities you engage in.

Set yourself up for success by eating a healthy breakfast (with plenty of protein!), getting at least thirty minutes of sun each day, going to bed at a decent hour, spending less time on your phone and more time moving your body.

Your period is an inflammatory process. This means that you may experience some discomfort in different parts of your body leading up to and during your period. This should not, however, keep you from school or from enjoying normal activities like sitting, sleeping, or going for a walk.

Making healthy choices between periods is key to avoiding extreme period pain and discomfort!

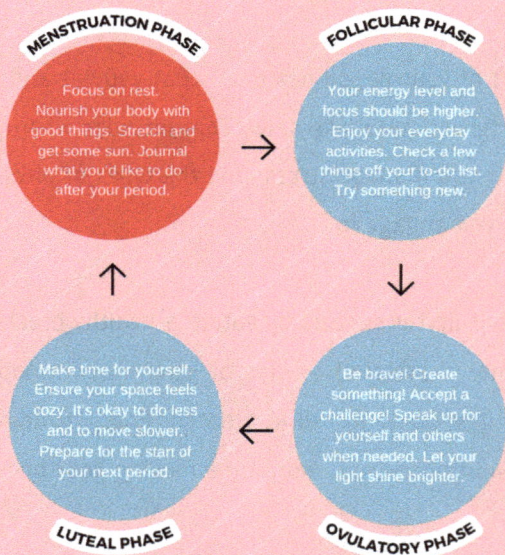

MENSTRUATION PHASE
Focus on rest. Nourish your body with good things. Stretch and get some sun. Journal what you'd like to do after your period.

FOLLICULAR PHASE
Your energy level and focus should be higher. Enjoy your everyday activities. Check a few things off your to-do list. Try something new.

LUTEAL PHASE
Make time for yourself. Ensure your space feels cozy. It's okay to do less and to move slower. Prepare for the start of your next period.

OVULATORY PHASE
Be brave! Create something! Accept a challenge! Speak up for yourself and others when needed. Let your light shine brighter.

The diagram above illustrates the different phases of your menstrual cycle and a few examples of ways you can care for your mind and body during each phase. There are no limitations here, but as I mentioned before, tune into your own body and monitor what you need as you move through each phase.

Food

Prioritize eating foods that give your body the vitamins and nutrients it needs to thrive. That means eating protein and veggies with every meal, swapping sweets for fruits, and adding healthy fats to your plate to reduce unhealthy cravings and keep you full. (See page 44.)

Take a look at your breakfast, your lunch, and your dinner plate each day. Observe what you see and decide what foods look the healthiest, then eat more of those. The same applies to your snack choices.

Drink

Hydrating with water is so important!

Sugary sodas and juices can zap your body of nutrients, leave you dehydrated, and increase your discomfort around your period. Trust me – you don't want that! Drinking more water than soda or caffeinated drinks will serve you well.

That's a promise.

Get creative and purchase a fun, refillable water bottle to carry in your bookbag and drink throughout the day.

If you need a little flavor in your water, add lemon or some other fruit, cucumber, or mint leaves.

Sleep

This one's tough because I know you might want to stay up late sometimes; but I also know what it's like to have a hard time waking up or wanting a nap in the middle of my period. This is no fun when there's work to do.

Prioritize good sleep habits now. That means not eating too close to bedtime, limiting your screen time in the evening, allowing yourself to get ready for bed as soon as you feel yourself winding down, and getting sun first thing in the morning.

Your body is smart! It knows when it's time to rest and when it's time to welcome a new day. Don't fight it. When your period comes around, you will be better because you are well-rested and in sync with your body's natural rhythms.

Stress Management

If you notice that you make unhealthy choices when you are having a bad day, then take note of that. Those unhealthy choices could look like oversleeping, not getting enough exercise, scrolling on your phone for too long, or eating too much candy.

A better way could include talking to a friend, spending time outdoors, listening to music, journaling, or helping your parent or guardian prepare dinner.

These are just a few examples of how you can manage stress in ways that support a healthy period and lifestyle.

Physical Activity

Your body was made to move!

As you continue to grow and develop, you will notice that your body feels better overall when you incorporate movement into your day. That is because exercise increases your happy hormones.

Happy hormones come in handy before and during your
period as they improve your mood and distract you from any
discomfort you might feel.

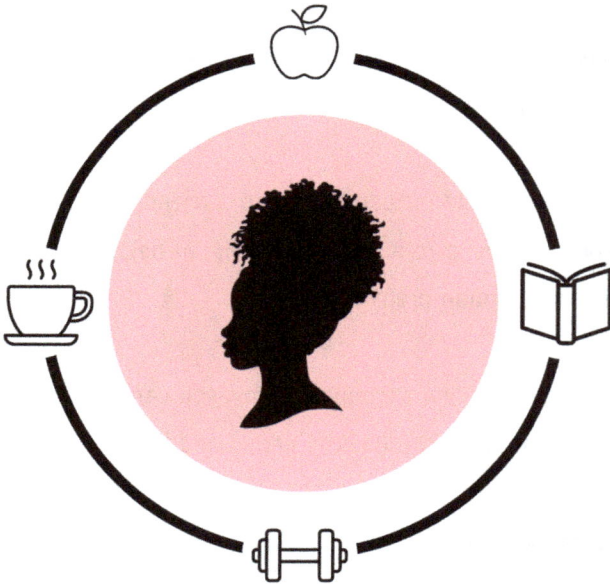

A Quick Note

Don't be anxious about any of the topics we covered in this
chapter. Refer back to it as you pick up on patterns in your
menstrual cycle, then focus on the topics that are most
relevant to you. Use your journal as a guide.

MY HEALTHY HABIT GOALS

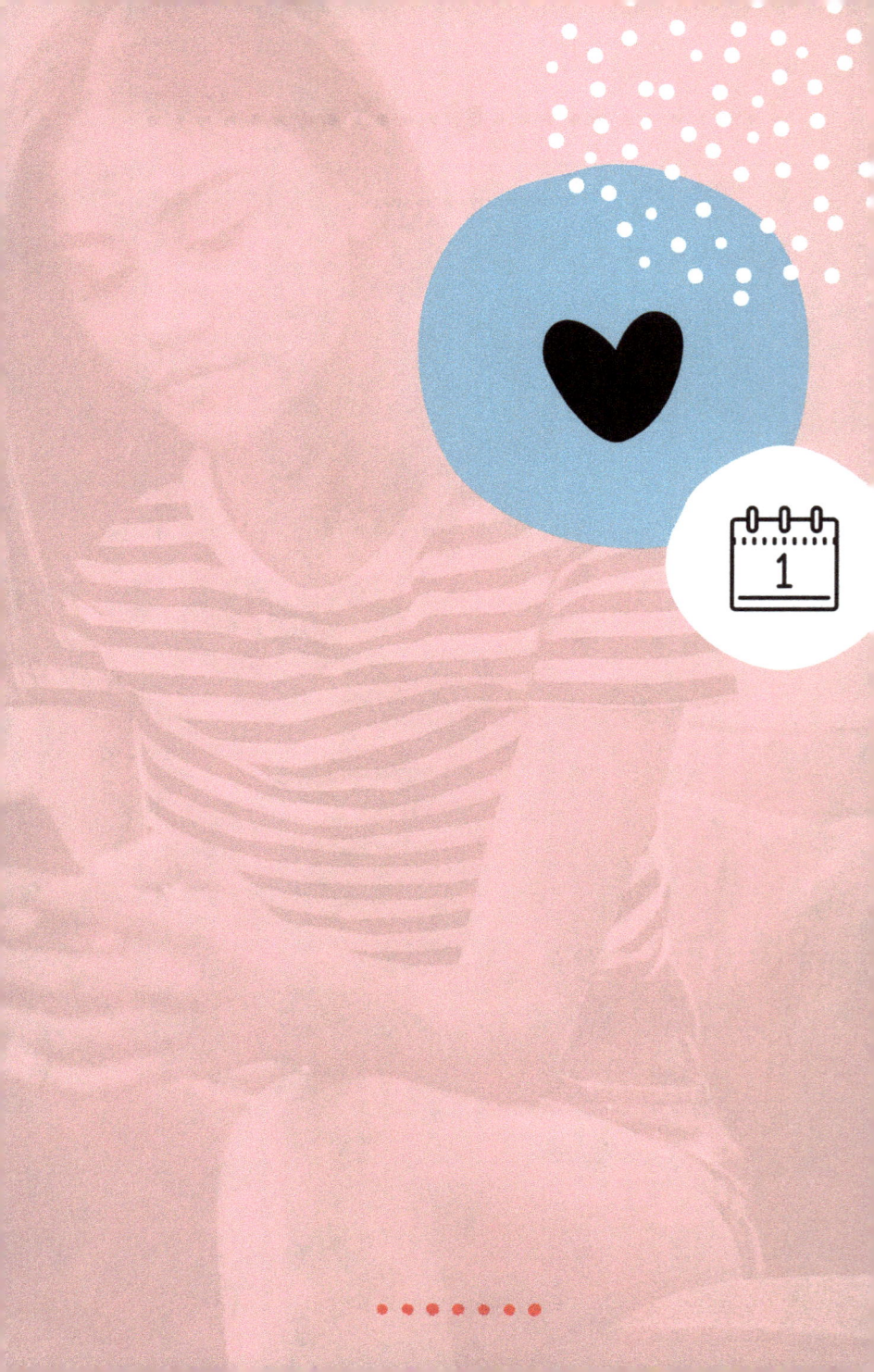

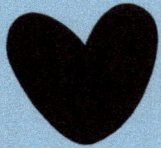

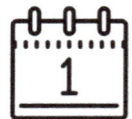

CHAPTER 7
Period Solutions

So when period problems arise, what do you do? I'm glad you asked!

Let me be clear: your period in and of itself is not a problem; however, some of the choices you make can create period-related problems - many of which can be avoided.

Let's talk about *Premenstrual Syndrome (PMS)*. PMS is a collection of physical and psychological symptoms that young girls and women experience about 2 to 7 days before the start of their period. If not addressed, these symptoms can severely affect your mood, focus, appetite, sleep, and even your appearance.

Here are a few of the most common symptoms and how to get through them:

Pain & Bloating

Period pain can include headaches, abdominal cramping, backaches, and digestive issues like diarrhea. To minimize period pain, drink plenty of water and limit your intake of sweets and refined carbohydrates (think packaged cookies and chips) - not just during your period, but daily, as this will reduce excess inflammation in your body.

Some discomfort is normal during your period, but it should not disrupt your life.

For example, you may experience some bloating during your period, but that's normal. If it makes you feel miserable, then that's a problem. To minimize bloating, stay away from salty foods, eat dark leafy greens (think spinach), and hydrate often. It is also a good idea to avoid foods and drinks that normally upset your tummy - even the slightest.

Pro tip: Hot herbal tea or a heating pad can be your best friends during this time. Request the help of an adult to prepare tea and to use a heating pad properly. If hot tea, heating pads, stretching, and warm baths don't reduce your period pain, then ask your parent(s) for some mild medicine.

Low Energy & Moodiness

If you find yourself feeling extra tired or moody, then follow the previous steps, incorporate sun and gentle movement into your day, and ensure you're getting a good night's rest (at least 8 hours).

Remember, it is okay to rest a little more during this time, especially in the days leading up to your period.

When you're not recharging, get some fresh air and make sure you're eating enough real food each day. That means limiting your caffeine and sugar intake, and eating meals. This will help you stabilize your blood sugar and avoid emotional roller coasters.

Some young girls experience *Premenstrual Dysphoric Disorder (PMDD)*, which is a severe mood disorder that affects their daily life. This may look like extreme sadness, anxiety, low energy, and a lot of anger. PMDD should be taken seriously and requires a diagnosis for treatment.

Other girls experience low energy because they lose more blood than they should, so keep an eye on that. (See page 47.)

Junk Food Cravings

Although you may feel the urge to eat junk food, don't overdo it, especially on an empty stomach! Eating a candy bar for lunch may feel good in the moment, but what your body needs most is protein, veggies, fruits, and healthy fats like avocados, pasture-raised eggs, and yogurt.

Real food can change your cravings and your period for the better. (See my food swaps below for inspiration.)

Eat your meals first; and if you're craving a sweet treat, grab some Lily's dark chocolate from the grocery store or bake something from scratch at home 🙂.

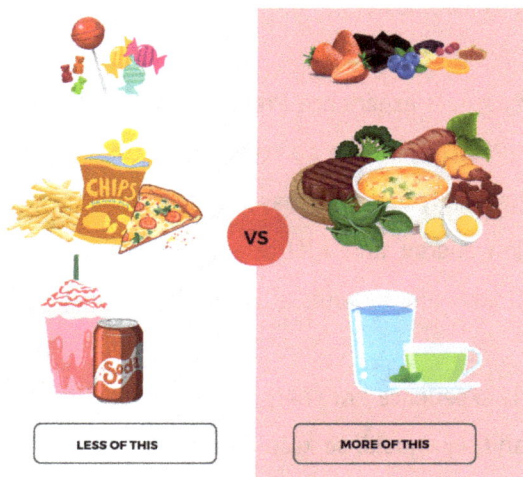

LESS OF THIS   VS   MORE OF THIS

Leaks & Odors

It may take a while to get a handle on this, but the best piece of advice I can give here is to purchase the right size period protection, change it often (every 3-4 hours), and follow the hygiene steps in Chapter 3.

It's okay to dismiss yourself every couple of hours to ensure your period protection is doing its job. **In no time, you will become an expert of your own body and develop healthy habits that keep leaks and odors under control.** You will also learn the art of readjusting your period protection to catch leaks where they most commonly occur.

Visit pages 53 and 56 of this book for more tips on maintaining freshness. You will smell your period blood from time to time, but neither you or anyone around you should smell it through your clothes.

It's okay to dismiss yourself every couple of hours to ensure your period protection is doing its job.

Period Acne

Pesky pimples and breakouts can be reduced by nourishing your body from the inside out! This starts with what you eat and drink on a daily basis, plus how you cleanse your face.

Don't underestimate the power of drinking water and eating well-balanced meals. **Your skin is counting on you to feed your body good things – to keep it clear, but most importantly, healthy.**

Over time, you will notice that your skin is happier when you limit sodas, fast food, and refined sugars in your diet.

Use a gentle, fragrance-free cleanser to wash your face regularly, and resist the temptation to pop pimples. You can follow up with a moisturizer, but beyond that, there's really no need to experiment with other skincare products.

Pro tip: blemish patches are available in a variety of fun shapes and colors - some of which can be worn discretely! They're great for healing pimples and serve as little reminders not to touch them.

Bleeding Between Periods, Heavy Periods, Long Periods, Missing Periods

If you find that you are bleeding between periods, bleeding too heavily (for example, soaking through pads every hour), or bleeding for too long (8 days or more), then you must take these things seriously. The same is true if your period goes missing for more than three months out of a year, after the first few years of your period.

You may notice some inconsistencies in the timing, flow, and length of your period early on; however, these things usually work themselves out as you grow.

Unfortunately, that's not always the case for all girls. This can make their periods extremely hard and points to other issues that should be checked out.

If your period remains unpredictable or disruptive, then take good notes and talk to an adult who will listen. They can work with you to look for clues and determine next steps.

If ever you find that your period is stressful in any way, or makes you feel anxious or sad, then talk to your doctor.

Despite what anyone might lead you to believe, a pain-free period is possible. Your period is not your enemy. Having a period is a completely normal, natural thing. It is working for you - not against you! Beautiful things will come from it, but you must remember to nourish your body and treat it well.

Think of your body as a strong, but delicate flower that needs good soil, water, and sun. Handle it with care from this day forward, from the inside out. Schedule rest days, take breaks, cry if you need to, think good thoughts about yourself, talk to someone you trust, pray.

Do what you need to do to feel like your best self, to continue blooming and becoming the woman God made you to be!

Your body will thank you, and it will show through your period.

My hope is that you feel empowered and capable of navigating your next periods with confidence. You have the information you need to handle any twists and turns, and potentially help others along the way.

Read this book over and over again, share it, and keep taking notes. (There's space on pages 69-71!)

Lastly, you will find additional information and resources on the next few pages. These include:

- Frequently asked questions
- A list of items to add to your period kit
- Period stories and anecdotes (for funsies!)
- Monthly calendar templates
- And more!

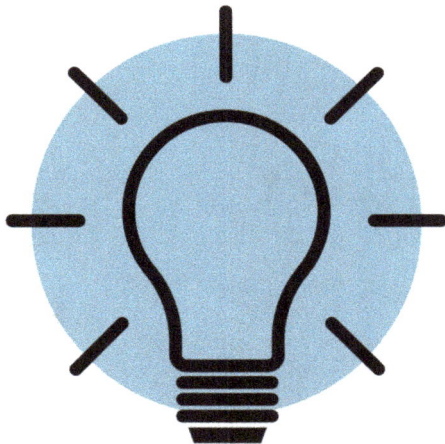

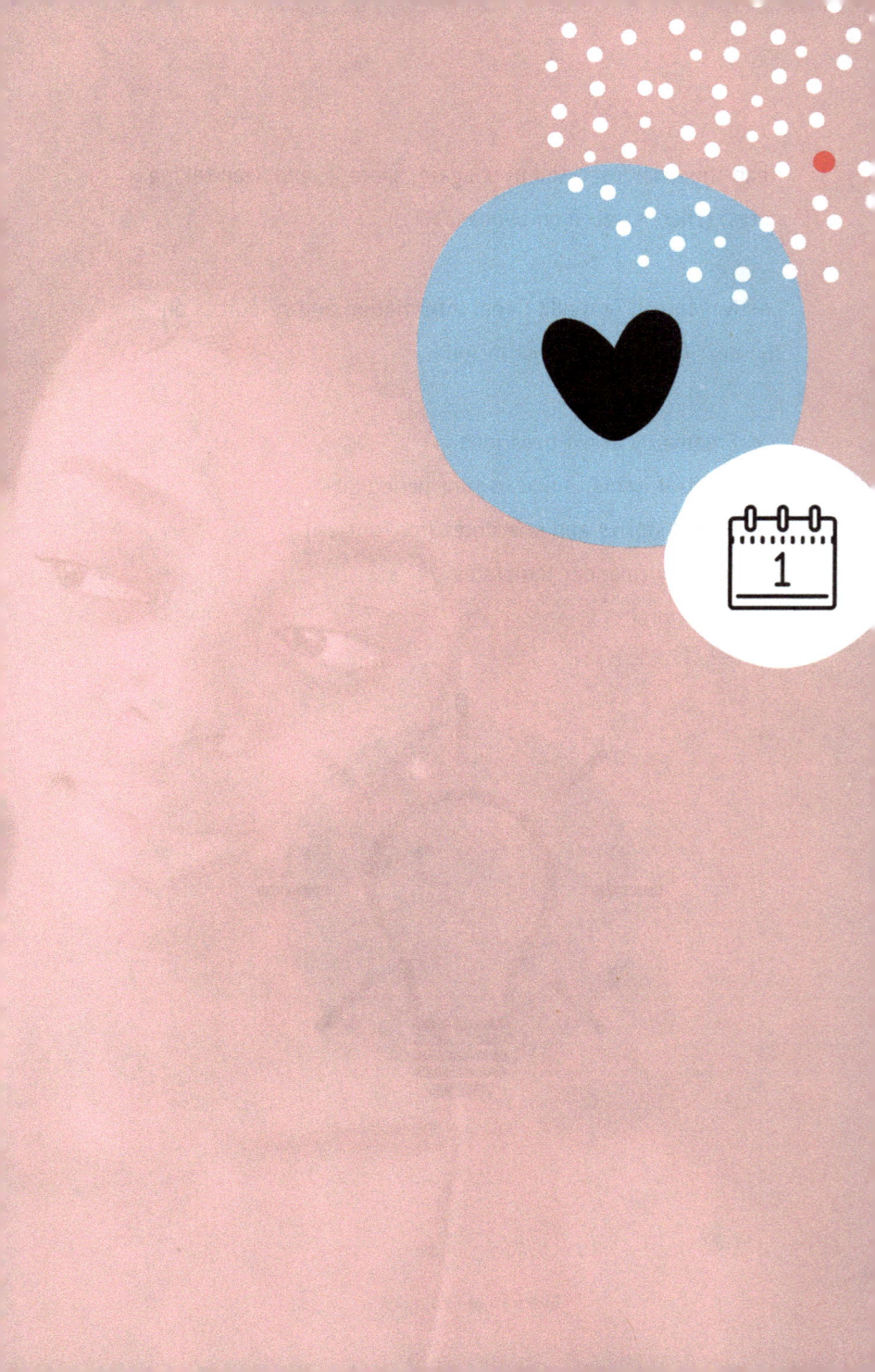

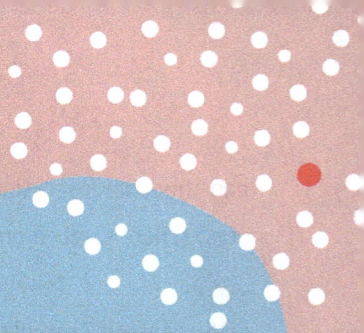

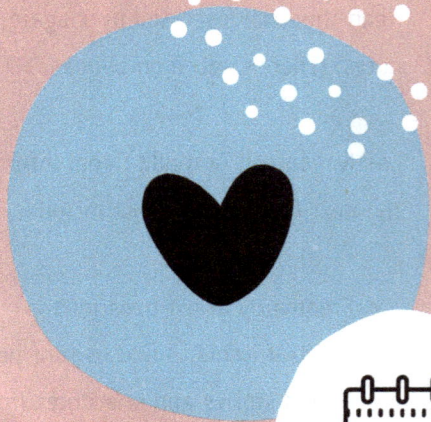

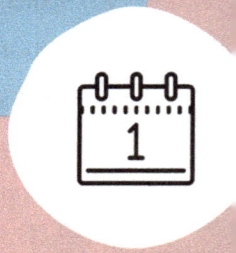

FAQs

How long should my period last? Your period can last anywhere from 2 to 7 days, but as you mature, it should last 3 to 7 days. In the first few years, the length may vary.

Can I exercise while I'm on my period? Yes. Light exercise such as walking and stretching is okay. Anything more than that might be excessive, but listen to what your body needs and rest more than you work out.

Can I go swimming while on my period? Yes, but with the right period protection, such as a tampon. This should be removed immediately after you swim. Period swimwear is also available. Remember, your period flow might be slower in the pool, but it does not go away. Do not swim in a pad.

Is it normal to experience cramping during my period? Light cramping is expected, but it should not be disruptive or debilitating (for example, you can't sit, stand, or complete normal tasks). No cramping is ideal.

What foods should I eat during my period? It is best to eat good sources of protein, dark green veggies, fruits, and healthy fats to stave off cravings and hunger. Warm soups and stews are great options.

Is it normal to experience diarrhea during my period? You may experience some digestive issues during your period, but much of this can be reduced by eliminating processed foods from your diet and anything that normally upsets your tummy or makes you poop a lot.

Can stress or anxiety change my period? Yes, increased stress or anxiety can make your period come later or not at all. Stress management is key (see Chapter 7). Incorporate breaks in your schedule and be sure to truly rest at night. Talk through your feelings with a friend or a parent when stressful situations arise.

Can hormonal birth control fix my period problems (e.g., cramps, acne, heavy bleeding, etc.)? No. Hormonal birth control keeps your body from doing what it naturally wants to do. This is no good for a growing girl. Healthy diet and lifestyle changes (see Chapter 6) are the way to go to fix most period problems.

Is bleeding between periods normal? No. This is called spotting or irregular, light bleeding that doesn't require a pad or tampon. If this issue persists, talk to your doctor.

Should my period be stinky? No, your period should not be stinky, but it may have a slight smell. If you notice a terrible odor during your period, follow the hygiene steps in Chapter 3. Wipe from front to back; wear clean and breathable cotton underwear; and shower regularly. If that doesn't help, then talk to an adult who can help.

How should I dress while I'm on my period? You can dress as normal, but until you fully understand the timing, flow, and duration of your period, I'd steer clear of any clothes that might make it difficult to hide leaks or bulky pads. For example, short shorts or white skirts may not be it.

I stained my sheets, towels, clothes, etc. Help! Rinse with cool water as soon as possible, then use soap to gently scrub the stain. If you need to use a stain remover, then apply that and let it sit for a few minutes before you rinse and place in the washer as normal. For tougher stains on light colored clothing or whites, spot treat with hydrogen peroxide or bleach with the help of an adult.

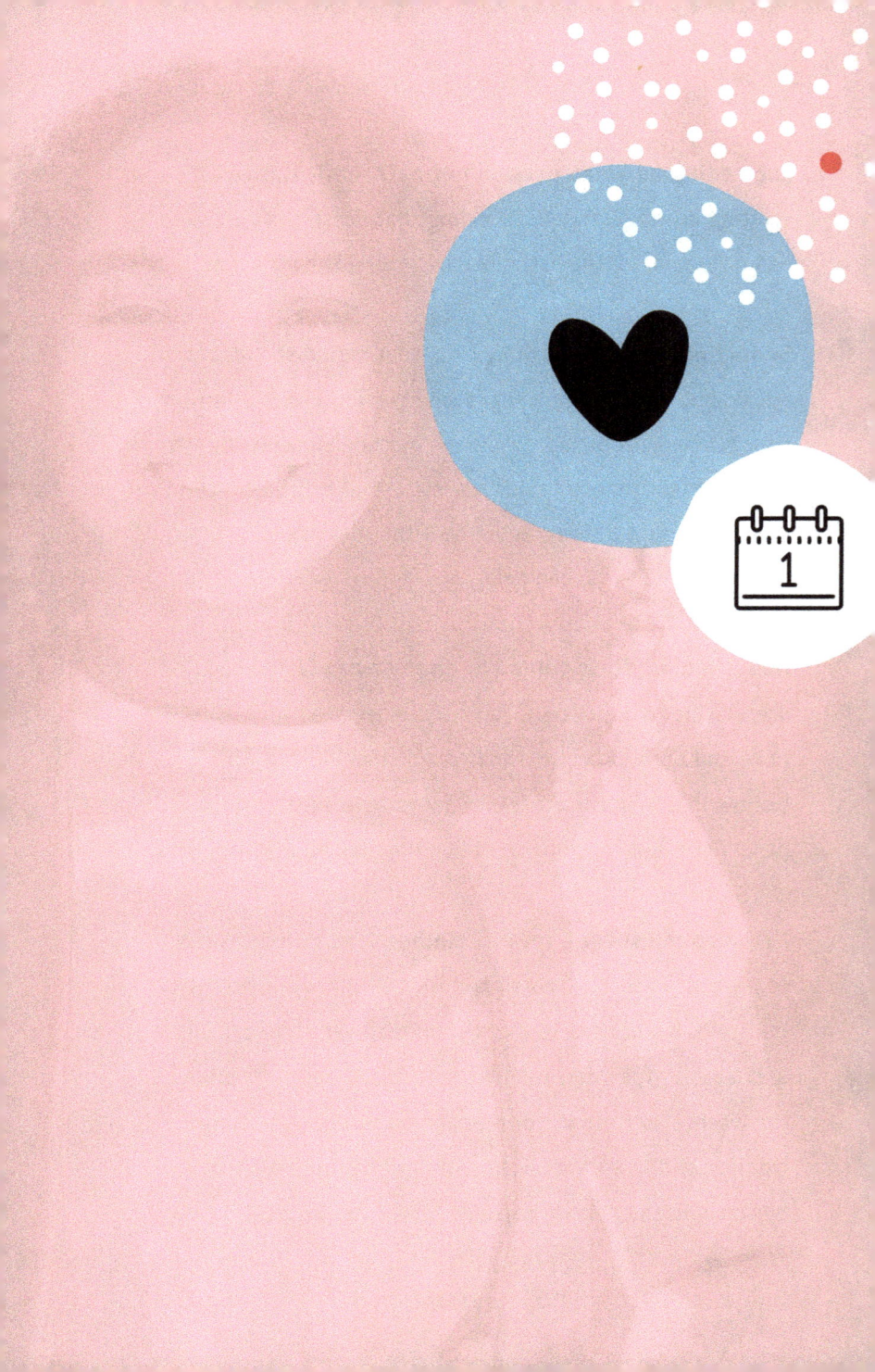

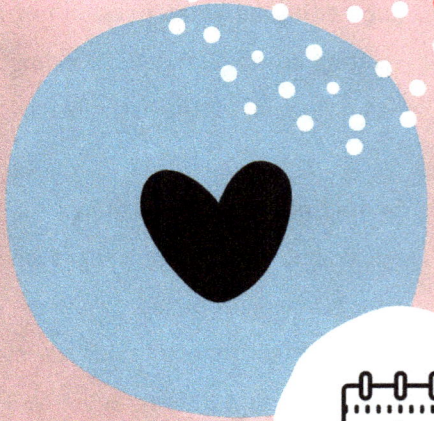

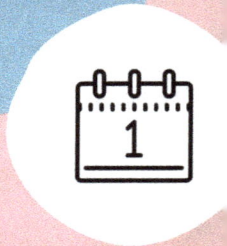

What to Add to Your Period Kit

Many of the items on this list can be added to your period kit for your on-the-go needs. Others can be stored in a cupboard for at-home use. Review the list, then build a small kit for your backpack!

Period protection

- 100% organic cotton pads, liners, and tampons
- Period panties for an extra layer of protection while sleeping or traveling

Period pain management

- Organic raspberry leaf tea and dandelion root tea
- Heating pad, hot water bottle, or ThermaCare wraps
- Magnesium flakes for bath time
- Ibuprofen - taken under parental supervision only! Never take pills from someone else.
- Castor oil packs - between periods only! Never apply while on your period.

Hygiene

- In the shower – gentle, fragrance-free soap for external cleansing only
- On the go – water wipes to freshen up, and hand sanitizer to kill germs on your hands before handling your period protection
- Spare 100% cotton underwear that's breathable and easy to clean. (Be sure to get the right size – nothing too tight or too big!)
- A small plastic bag to store stained undies until you get home to wash them

Extras

- Travel size deodorant
- Tide To Go Stick to treat stains
- Essential oil roller in lavender or another calming scent to manage stress
- Blemish patches to cover pimples

Keep your kit ready and accessible! If someone you know needs period supplies, don't be afraid to offer up what you're not using 🙂.

My Period Kit

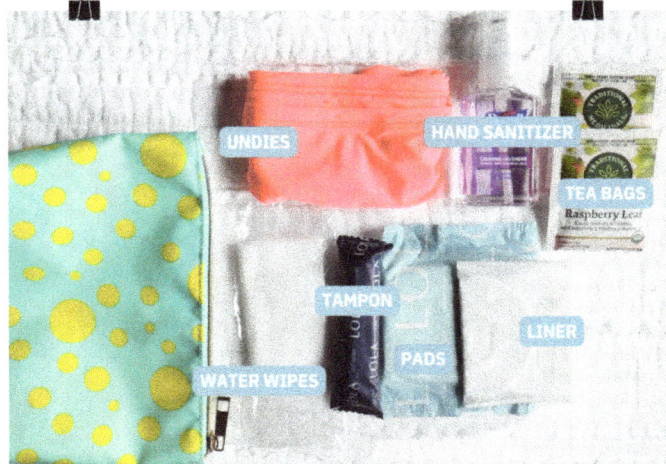

UNDIES · HAND SANITIZER · TEA BAGS Raspberry Leaf · TAMPON · PADS · LINER · WATER WIPES

This is what I keep in my on-the-go period kit, but you can add whatever you'd like to yours! Follow me on Instagram @everypage.mhl for a peek at my favorite things!

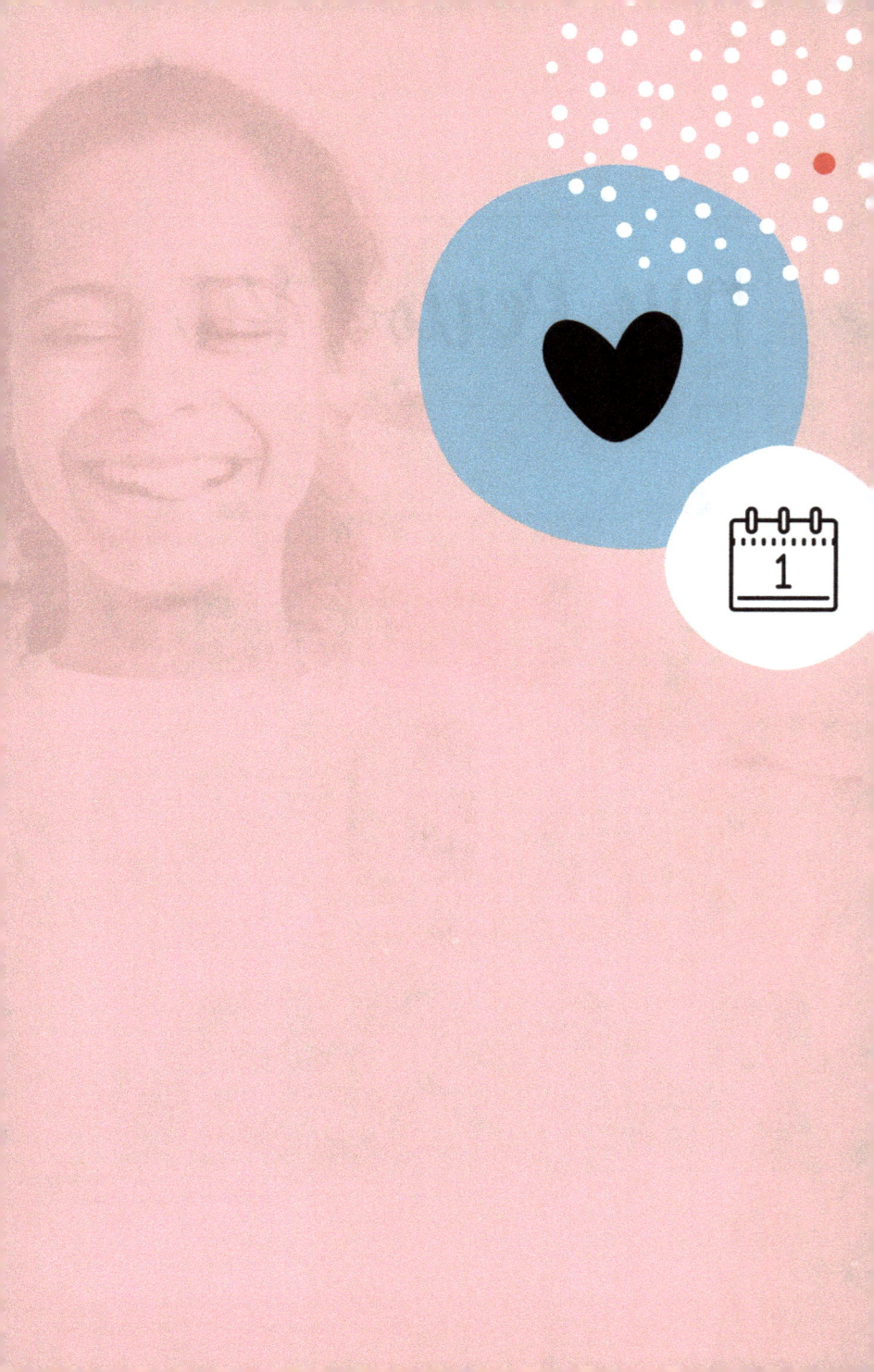

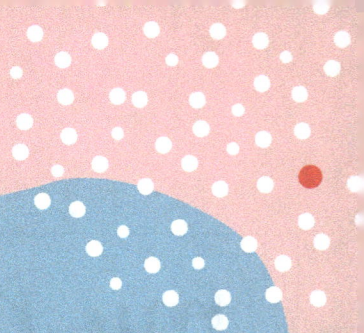

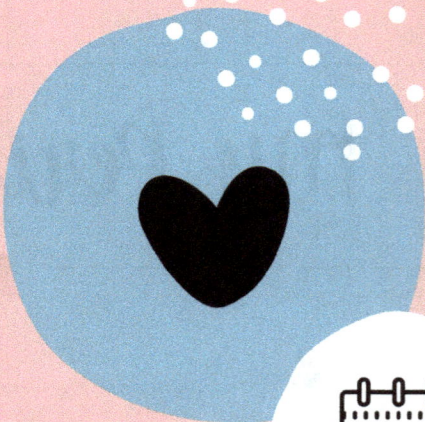

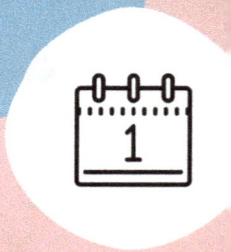

Period Stories

"I was about 13 and in the 7th grade enjoying gym class with my friends. I'm running around when my guy best friend comes up to me and pulls me to the side to tell me I messed up my pants. I didn't know what he was referring to until it dawned on me, I finally got my period. He was so matter of fact, I couldn't be embarrassed. I totally appreciated him for that." – Toni

---

"I was trying to discreetly tell my parents that we needed to stop by the store on the way home because I needed some pads. My brother, who was around 10 at the time, asked why we had to stop. My dad, an OBGYN, decided to use it as a teaching moment [and] told my brother that I was on my period and needed pads. My brother's response, "yeah but we have band aids at home, how bad can it be?" – Michelle

"I threw out an alarming number of tampons (as a teen and a young adult) trying to figure out how to consistently insert one the right way. Sometimes I would get it. Most times, I wouldn't. Fast forward a couple of decades and I finally figured it out. In that moment, I felt so accomplished. Moral of the story: go at your own pace. You have time." - Dee

---

"The craziest thing about a period is when it bubbles up the back of your undies and misses the entire pad. I was in junior high school when this first happened to me and I was completely dumbfounded. From then on, I wore an extra pad until longer ones came along." - Sharon

---

"One of the best feelings in the world is unexpectedly starting your period, but remembering that you have a spare pad or tampon in your bag or in your car! Even better when you're able to save the day by sharing that spare with a friend in need. Girl code for the win!" - Erica

MY PERIOD STORY

DATE: _____

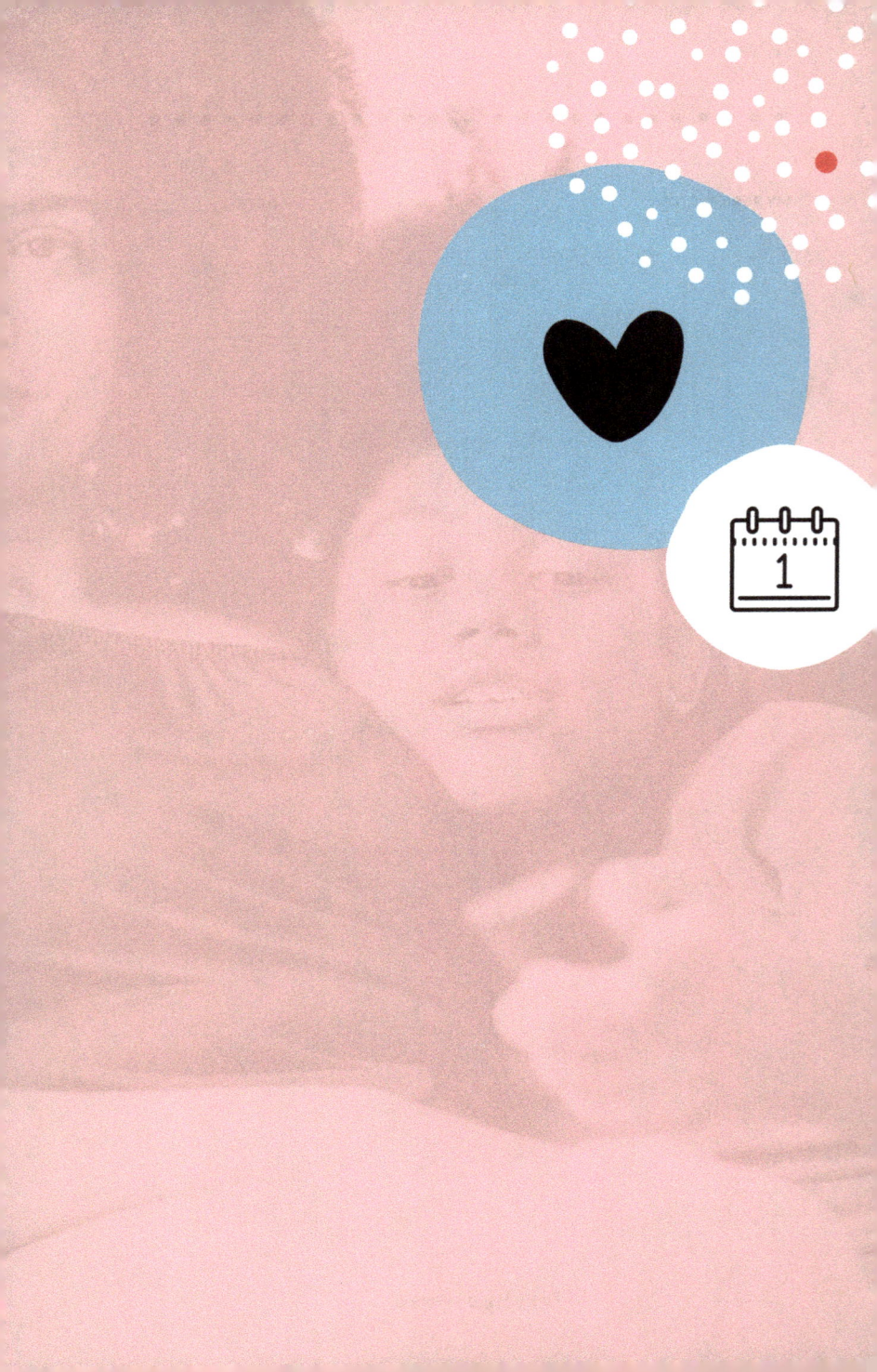

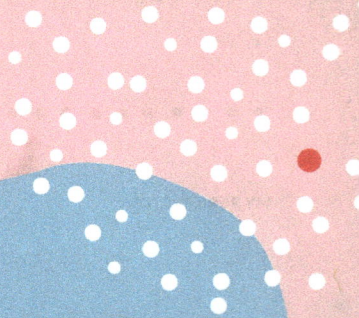

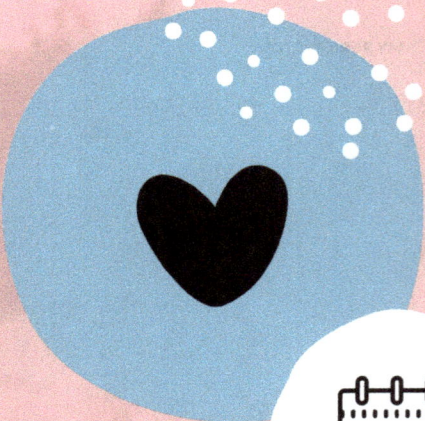

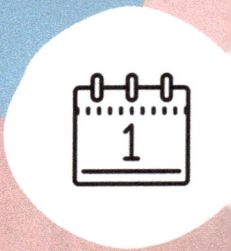

A Message for Parents

After reading this book, I hope you feel inspired to continue to engage in healthy conversations about periods. It is possible to talk to young girls about their period in ways that build them up and prepare them for the road ahead.

Periods and period problems should not be taboo topics. The more you express care and respect in these regards, the better. That means offering support and avoiding crude jokes and insensitive comments about periods.

As a parent (or guardian), you can help increase awareness around periods without diving too deep into subject matter that may not be age-appropriate. You can also be an advocate and help find solutions when period problems arise.

Menstruation is a broad topic, so give yourself time to learn alongside the little ladies in your life, at a pace that feels comfortable for them and your family.

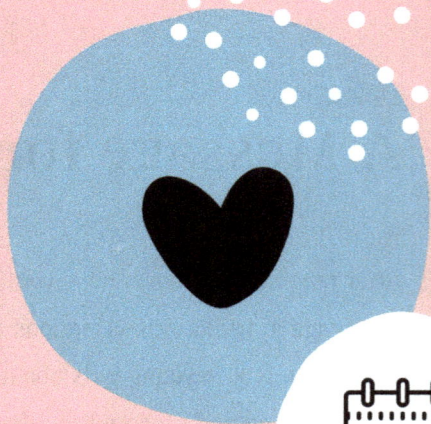

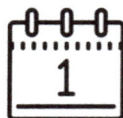

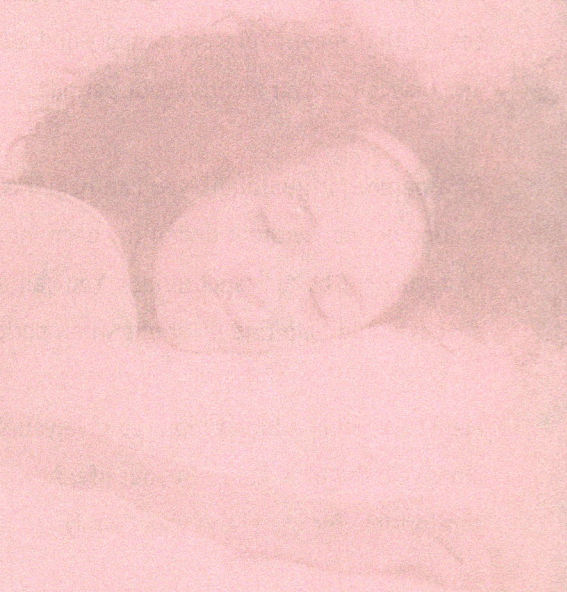

MONTHLY PERIOD CALENDAR (EXAMPLE)

October

S	M	T	W	T	F	S
1	2	3	4	5	6	7
8 ☹	9 ☹	10 ①	11 ②	12 ③	13 ④	14 ⑤
15 ☺	16 ☺	17 ☺	18	19	20	21
22	23	24	25	26	27	28
29	30	31				

Oct 8: I felt a bit sad
Oct 9: I didn't get enough sleep
Oct 11-12: My period flow was heavy

☺ GOOD DAY ☹ NOT-SO-GOOD DAY 🔴 BLEEDING DAY

MONTHLY PERIOD CALENDAR (EXAMPLE)

November

S	M	T	W	T	F	S
			1	2	3	4
5 ☹	6 ☹	7 ☹	8 ①	9 ②	10 ③	11 ④
12 ⑤	13 ☺	14 ☺	15 ☺	16	17	18
19	20	21	22	23	24	25
26	27	28	29	30		

Nov 5: I didn't want to go to school
Nov 6-7: I slept through my alarm!
Nov 10: My period flow was much lighter

☺ GOOD DAY ☹ NOT-SO-GOOD DAY 🔴 BLEEDING DAY

MONTHLY PERIOD CALENDAR

S	M	T	W	T	F	S

🙂 GOOD DAY 🙁 NOT-SO-GOOD DAY 🔴 BLEEDING DAY

MONTHLY PERIOD CALENDAR

S	M	T	W	T	F	S

🙂 GOOD DAY 🙁 NOT-SO-GOOD DAY 🔴 BLEEDING DAY

MONTHLY PERIOD CALENDAR

S	M	T	W	T	F	S

☺ GOOD DAY ☹ NOT-SO-GOOD DAY ● BLEEDING DAY

MONTHLY PERIOD CALENDAR

S	M	T	W	T	F	S

☺ GOOD DAY ☹ NOT-SO-GOOD DAY ● BLEEDING DAY

MONTHLY PERIOD CALENDAR

S	M	T	W	T	F	S

🙂 GOOD DAY 🙁 NOT-SO-GOOD DAY 🔴 BLEEDING DAY

MONTHLY PERIOD CALENDAR

S	M	T	W	T	F	S

🙂 GOOD DAY 🙁 NOT-SO-GOOD DAY 🔴 BLEEDING DAY

NOTES

NOTES

NOTES

Index

The Author

Teri Durden, IMH-C, also known as "The Period Planner," is the founder of Every Page Menstrual Health Literacy. She holds a M.S. in Community & Regional Planning, but mostly enjoys helping women plan for consistent, non-disruptive, and ovulatory periods. Certified by the Institute for Menstrual Health, Teri is a Christ-follower, lover of learning, and believer in the power of dark green veggies.

FIND ME

Email :
teri@everypage.blog

Website :
everypage.blog

Instagram Handle:
@theperiodplanner

Instagram Handle:
@everypage.mhl

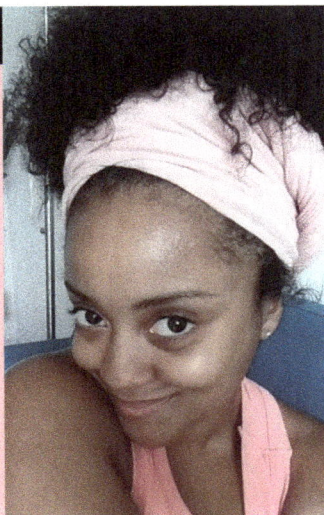

www.ingramcontent.com/pod-product-compliance
Lightning Source LLC
Chambersburg PA
CBHW060256030426
42335CB00014B/1719